The Mind-Body Blueprint

Unlocking the Secrets to Optimal Health and Wellness

Floyd W. Kent

DISCLAIMER

TABLE OF CONTENT

CHAPTER 5

CHAPTER 6

INTRODUCTION

"Welcome to 'The Mind-Body Blueprint: Unlocking the Secrets to Optimal Health and Wellness.' In this book, we will explore the powerful connection between the mind and body, and how understanding and harnessing this connection can lead to optimal health and wellness.

Throughout this book, you will learn about the latest scientific research on the mind-body connection, and how it can be applied to improve physical and mental health. We will discuss the importance of nutrition, physical activity, stress management, and mindfulness in achieving optimal health and wellness.

You will also learn about the benefits of a holistic approach to health and wellness, and how to create a personalized mind-body blueprint that takes into account your unique needs and preferences.

This book is designed for anyone who is looking to improve their physical and mental well-being. Whether you're looking to lose weight, reduce stress, or improve your overall health, this book will provide you with the knowledge and tools you need to achieve your goals.

So, let's begin our journey towards optimal health and wellness, and unlock the secrets of the mind-body connection.

CHAPTER 1

UNDERSTANDING THE MIND-BODY CONNECTION

"Understanding the Mind-Body Connection" refers to the idea that the mind and body are closely interconnected and that one can affect the other. The concept of the mind-body connection has been studied and discussed in many fields, including psychology, medicine, and philosophy. It suggests that the mind and body are not separate entities, but rather work together in a complex interplay.

One aspect of the mind-body connection is the idea that our thoughts, emotions, and beliefs can have a direct impact on our physical health. For example, stress and anxiety can lead to physical symptoms such as headaches, muscle tension, and an increased risk of illness.

Conversely, physical activities such as yoga and meditation can help to reduce stress and improve overall health.

Another aspect of the mind-body connection is the idea that physical conditions can also affect our mental and emotional well-being. For example, chronic pain can lead to depression and anxiety, while certain medical conditions such as autoimmune disorders can have a significant impact on a person's quality of life.

Understanding the mind-body connection is important for developing effective treatments for both physical and mental health conditions. It suggests that a holistic approach that addresses both the mind and the body is necessary for optimal health and well-being. This can include therapies such as cognitive-behavioral therapy, mindfulness practices, and physical exercise, as well as conventional medical treatments.

Understanding the mind-body connection is crucial for promoting and maintaining good health. It highlights the importance of considering the whole person - mind, body, and spirit - when addressing health issues, and encourages the integration of different approaches to healing and wellness

THE SCIENCE OF THE MIND-BODY CONNECTION

The science of the mind-body connection refers to the relationship between our mental and emotional states and our physical health. Research has shown that our thoughts, emotions, and beliefs can have a direct impact on our physiological processes and overall well-being.

One of the key ways in which the mind and body are connected is through the nervous system. The nervous system is responsible for communicating information between the brain and the rest of the body. When we experience stress, for example, our brain sends signals to the body to release stress hormones such as cortisol and adrenaline, which can cause physical reactions such as increased heart rate and blood pressure.

Another important aspect of the mind-body connection is the role of the immune system. Our immune system is responsible for fighting off illness and disease, and research has shown that stress and negative emotions can weaken the immune system, making us more susceptible to illness. On the other hand, positive emotions and relaxation can strengthen the immune system.

The mind-body connection also plays a role in the development and management of chronic conditions such as heart disease, diabetes, and autoimmune disorders. Studies have shown that stress and negative emotions can worsen these conditions, while relaxation and positive emotions can improve symptoms.

The science of the mind-body connection demonstrates the intricate relationship between our mental and emotional states and our physical health, and highlights the importance of addressing both aspects of well-being in order to achieve optimal health and wellness.

HOW OUR THOUGHS AND EMOTIONS AFFECT OUR PHYSICAL HEALTH

Our thoughts and emotions can have a significant impact on our physical health. Studies have shown that there is a strong connection between our mental and emotional states and our physiological processes.

One way in which our thoughts and emotions affect our physical health is through the release of stress hormones. When we experience stress or negative emotions, our brain sends signals to the body to release hormones such as cortisol and adrenaline, which can lead to physical reactions such as increased heart rate and blood pressure. These reactions can have negative effects on our health over time if the stress is chronic, and can contribute to conditions such as heart disease and diabetes.

Another way in which our thoughts and emotions affect our physical health is through the immune system. Stress and negative emotions can weaken the immune system, making us more susceptible to illness. On the other hand, positive emotions and relaxation can strengthen the immune system, helping to fight off illness and disease.

Our thoughts and emotions can also affect our physical health through the placebo effect. This is the phenomenon where a person's belief in a treatment or medication can cause them to feel better, even if the treatment or medication is not actually effective. Similarly, negative thoughts and beliefs can lead to the nocebo effect, where a person's belief in negative outcomes can lead to them experiencing negative side effects.

Our thoughts and emotions can affect our physical health through our behavior. Negative thoughts and emotions can lead to unhealthy behaviors such as overeating, smoking, and lack of physical activity, which can contribute to chronic health conditions. On the other hand, positive thoughts and emotions can lead to healthy behaviors such as eating well, exercising, and getting enough sleep, which can promote good health.

IDENTIFYING AND PRIORITIZING YOUR NEEDS.

Identifying and prioritizing your needs is an essential step in creating an effective self-care routine. Self-care is the practice of taking care of your physical, mental, and emotional well-being in order to maintain or improve your overall health.

To identify your needs, you can start by taking inventory of your current state of well-being. Consider how you are feeling physically, mentally, and emotionally. Are you feeling stressed, exhausted, or overwhelmed? Are you struggling with a specific health condition or chronic pain? Are you feeling lonely or disconnected? These are all important factors to take into consideration when identifying your needs.

Once you have identified your needs, you can then prioritize them based on their level of urgency and importance. For example, if you are dealing with a chronic health condition, you may want to prioritize self-care activities that help manage that condition, such as exercise and stress management techniques. If you are feeling lonely or disconnected, you may want to prioritize self-care activities that help you connect with others, such as socializing or joining a group or club.

IMPLEMENTING A SELF-CARE ROUTINE

Implementing a self-care routine is the next step after identifying and prioritizing your needs. The key to creating an effective self-care routine is to make it sustainable

and realistic. This means that you should choose self-care activities that you enjoy and that you can realistically fit into your daily or weekly schedule.

Here are some examples of self-care activities:

1. Physical self-care: regular exercise, healthy eating, getting enough sleep, and taking care of your skin.

2. Mental self-care: meditation, journaling, reading, and practicing mindfulness.

3. Emotional self-care: practicing gratitude, spending time with loved ones, and doing activities that make you happy.

4. Spiritual self-care: practicing a religion, connecting with nature, and engaging in activities that bring you a sense of peace and purpose.

It's also important to make self-care a regular part of your routine, instead of something you do occasionally. Scheduling self-care activities into your calendar and set reminder can be helpful.

Remember that self-care is not a luxury but a necessity, and taking time to care for yourself can help improve your overall well-being.

CHAPTER 3

NUTRITION AND THE MIND-BODY CONNECTION

THE ROLE OF NUTRITION IN PHYSICAL AND MENTAL HEALTH

The role of nutrition in physical and mental health is well-established. Proper nutrition is essential for maintaining good health and preventing chronic diseases. Eating a diet rich in nutrient-dense foods can help to promote optimal physical and mental health, while a poor diet can contribute to a wide range of health problems.

Nutrition plays a key role in maintaining a healthy body weight, building and repairing muscle and bone, and providing the energy needed for physical activity. Eating a healthy diet can also help to prevent chronic diseases such as heart disease, diabetes, and certain types of cancer.

Nutrition also plays a key role in mental health. Studies have shown that a diet high in fruits, vegetables, whole grains, and lean protein sources can lead to better mental health outcomes, while a diet high in processed foods,

sugar, and saturated fat can contribute to poor mental health.

THE BEST FOOD FOR OPTIMAL HEALTH AND WELLNESS

The best foods for optimal health and wellness include nutrient-dense options such as:

1. Fruits and vegetables: These provide a wide range of vitamins,

minerals, antioxidants, and fiber that are essential for good health.

2. Whole grains: Whole grains provide important nutrients such as B vitamins, minerals, and fiber.

3. Lean protein: Lean protein sources such as fish, poultry, and legumes provide important nutrients such as amino acids, iron, and zinc.

Healthy fats: Healthy fats such as those found in nuts, seeds, avocado, and olive oil provide important nutrients such as omega-3 fatty acids and vitamin E.

HOW TO CREATE BALANCED AND NOURISHING DIET

To create a balanced and nourishing diet, it's important to include a variety of nutrient-dense foods from all food groups in your diet, and to limit processed foods, added sugars, and saturated fats. A balanced diet should include:

Fruits and vegetables: Aim for at least 5 servings of fruits and vegetables per day.

Whole grains: Choose whole grains such as quinoa, brown rice, or whole wheat bread instead of refined grains.

Lean protein: Incorporate lean protein sources such as fish, poultry, and legumes into your diet.

Healthy fats: Include healthy fats such as those found in nuts, seeds, avocado, and olive oil in your diet.

It's also important to pay attention to portion sizes and to eat until you're satisfied but not overly full. Additionally, drinking enough water and limiting sugary drinks can also be beneficial for your diet.

CHAPTER 4

EXERCISE AND THE MIND-BODY CONNECTION

THE BENEFITS OF PHYSICAL ACTIVITIES

The benefits of physical activity are well-established, and regular exercise is an important aspect of maintaining good health. Some of the key benefits of physical activity include:

1. Improving cardiovascular health: Exercise improves heart and lung function, helping to lower the risk of heart disease and stroke.

2. Strengthening muscles and bones: Exercise helps to build and maintain muscle and bone mass, which can help to prevent conditions such as osteoporosis.

3. Managing weight: Regular exercise can help to maintain a

healthy body weight and reduce the risk of obesity.

4.   Improving mental health: Exercise has been shown to reduce symptoms of depression and anxiety, and improve overall mental well-being.

HOW TO CREATE AN EXCERCISE ROUTINE THAT WORKS FOR YOU

To create an exercise routine that works for you, it's important to consider your personal preferences and goals. Some people prefer to exercise alone, while others prefer to exercise with friends or in a group setting. Some people prefer to exercise outside, while others prefer to exercise indoors. Some people prefer high-intensity activities, while others prefer low-impact activities.

It's also important to consider your current fitness level and to start with a level of intensity that is appropriate for you. As you become more fit, you can gradually increase the intensity of your exercise routine.

When creating your exercise routine, it's also important to consider your schedule and to make sure that you have enough time to exercise on a regular basis. It can be helpful to schedule your exercise routine into your calendar, just like any other appointment.

THE RELATIONSHIP BETWEEN EXERCISE AND MENTAL HEALTH

The relationship between exercise and mental health is well-established. Regular exercise has been shown to reduce symptoms of depression and anxiety, and improve overall mental well-being. Exercise can help to release endorphins, which are chemicals in the brain that can improve mood and reduce feelings of stress and anxiety. Additionally, exercise can also help to improve sleep, which can further improve mental well-being.

Exercise can also help to improve self-esteem, boost confidence, and increase feelings of self-worth. Additionally, exercise can also serve as a form of stress relief and can help to reduce feelings of stress and anxiety.

It's important to note that the relationship between exercise and mental health is a two-way street. Poor mental health can make it harder to stick to an exercise routine, and this can further deteriorate mental health. It's important to find a balance and make sure to take care of both your physical and mental health.

CHAPTER 5

STRESS MANAGEMENT AND THE MIND-BODY CONNECTION

THE EFFECT OF STRESS ON THE BODY

The effects of stress on the body can be wide-ranging and can have both short-term and long-term consequences on one's physical and mental health. Stress activates the body's "fight or flight" response, which can cause a wide range of physical symptoms such as increased heart rate, blood pressure, and muscle tension. These symptoms can be temporary and can dissipate once the stressor is removed, but if stress is chronic, it can take a toll on the body over time.

Chronic stress can increase the risk of developing chronic health conditions such as heart disease, diabetes, and autoimmune disorders. It can also lead to a weakened immune system, making the body more susceptible to illness and disease.

Chronic stress can lead to physical symptoms such as headaches, fatigue, and muscle pain, as well as mental health issues such as depression, anxiety, and insomnia.

DIFFERENT TECHNIQUES FOR MANAGING STRESS

Managing stress is important for both physical and mental well-being. There are many different techniques for managing stress, including:

1. Relaxation techniques: Relaxation techniques such as deep breathing, meditation, and yoga can help to reduce muscle

tension and lower heart rate, blood pressure, and stress hormone levels.

2. Exercise: Regular physical activity can help to reduce stress by releasing endorphins, which are chemicals in the brain that can improve mood and reduce feelings of stress and anxiety.

3. Time management: Managing time effectively can help to reduce stress by ensuring that you have enough time to complete tasks

and by prioritizing important tasks.

4. Social support: Having a strong social support network can help to reduce stress by providing a source of emotional support and a sounding board for concerns.

HOW TO CREATE A STRESS MANAGEMENT PLAN

Creating a stress management plan can be an effective way to manage stress. A stress management plan should include a combination of different techniques that work best for you, such as:

1. Identifying triggers: Identify the things that trigger stress in your

life and try to avoid them as much as possible

2. Prioritizing self-care: Make self-care activities such as exercise, healthy eating, and getting enough sleep a priority.

3. Scheduling relaxation time: Set aside time each day for relaxation and stress-reduction activities such as deep breathing, yoga, or meditation.

4. Building a support system: Build a support system of friends and

family that you can turn to for emotional support when you're feeling stressed.

5. Seeking professional help: If stress continues to be a problem, consider seeking professional help from a therapist, counselor, or physician.

It's important to remember that stress is a normal part of life, but chronic stress can have negative effects on physical and mental health. By creating a stress management plan, you can take a proactive approach to managing stress and improve your overall well-being.

CHAPTER 6

MINDFULNESS AND THE BODY-MIND CONNECTION

UNDERSTANDING MINDFULNESS

Understanding mindfulness is the practice of being present and engaged in the current moment, without judgment. It involves paying attention to your thoughts, feelings, and physical sensations in a non-judgmental way.

Mindfulness is often associated with meditation and other contemplative practices, but it can also be practiced in daily activities such as walking, eating, and doing household chores.

Understanding mindfulness is the practice of being present and engaged in the current moment, without judgment. It involves paying attention to your thoughts, feelings, and physical sensations in a non-judgmental way. Mindfulness is often associated with meditation and other contemplative practices, but it can also be practiced in daily activities such as walking, eating, and doing household chores.

The goal of mindfulness is to increase awareness and acceptance of the present moment, which can help to reduce stress, improve mental well-being and physical health. Mindfulness helps to reduce negative thoughts and emotions by allowing individuals to observe them without judgment, and instead, focus on the present moment.

Mindfulness practices include:

Meditation: Sitting quietly and focusing on the breath, an object, or a guided meditation.

Mindful breathing: Paying attention to the breath as it goes in and out of the body

Mindful movement: such as yoga and tai chi

Body scan: Paying attention to each part of the body and how it feels

Loving-kindness meditation: Sending kind and compassionate thoughts to oneself and others

It's important to note that mindfulness is not about clearing the mind of thoughts but about observing thoughts and emotions without judgment, and returning to the present moment. Mindfulness is a skill that can be developed with regular practice, and it can be beneficial for both physical and mental well-being.

Understanding mindfulness is the practice of being present and engaged in the current moment, without judgment. It is the ability to pay attention to the present moment, in a non-reactive and non-judgmental way, and it can be cultivated through various techniques such as meditation, yoga, and mindful breathing. Mindfulness is often associated with Eastern spiritual traditions such as Buddhism, but it has become increasingly popular in Western cultures as a means of improving mental and physical health.

Mindfulness can be practiced in any moment, whether it's during a formal meditation session, a yoga class, or in daily activities such as walking, eating, or even washing dishes. The goal of mindfulness is to cultivate awareness of one's thoughts, feelings, and physical sensations in the present moment, and to observe them without judgment.

The practice of mindfulness can bring many benefits, such as:

1. Reducing stress and anxiety

2. Improving emotional regulation

3. Enhancing focus and concentration

4.Improving physical health and well-being

5. Improving relationships

6. Boosting creativity

Improving decision-making

It's important to note that mindfulness is a skill that takes practice, and it may be difficult to stay focused and present in the moment at first, but with consistent practice, it becomes easier to stay present in the moment and the benefits can be significant. Mindfulness practices can be incorporated into one's daily routine and can be adapted to fit personal needs and preferences

THE SCIENCE OF MINDFULNESS

The science of mindfulness is the study of the cognitive and physiological effects of mindfulness practices on the brain and body. Research has shown that mindfulness practices such as meditation can have a positive effect on mental and physical health. For example, studies have shown that mindfulness practices can reduce symptoms of depression and anxiety, improve attention and focus, and lower blood pressure and heart rate.

The science of mindfulness refers to the study of the cognitive and physiological effects of mindfulness practices on the brain and body. Research on

mindfulness has been growing in recent years and has provided a deeper understanding of the mechanisms through which mindfulness can improve mental and physical health.

One of the key ways in which mindfulness practices such as meditation can affect the brain is through changes in brain activity and structure. Studies have shown that regular mindfulness practices can lead to increased activity in the prefrontal cortex, which is involved in attention and decision-making, and decreased activity in the amygdala, which is involved in the stress response. Additionally, studies have also shown that mindfulness practices can lead to increased gray matter in the prefrontal cortex, which is associated with better cognitive function and emotional regulation.

Research has also shown that mindfulness practices can have positive effects on physical health. For example, studies have shown that mindfulness practices can lower blood pressure and heart rate, reduce chronic pain, and improve immune function. Additionally, mindfulness practices have been shown to reduce symptoms of mental health conditions such as depression and anxiety.

The benefits of mindfulness are not limited to adults, mindfulness practices have been adapted to children and adolescents, and research has shown that it can be effective in reducing symptoms of anxiety and depression, and improve overall well-being and cognitive function in children.

It's important to note that the research on the science of mindfulness is still ongoing, but the current evidence suggests that mindfulness practices can have a positive impact on both mental and physical health. Incorporating mindfulness into daily routine and practicing regularly can lead to measurable benefits on one's well-being.

HOW TO INCORPORATE MINDFULNESS INTO YOUR DAILY ROUTINE

Incorporating mindfulness into your daily routine can be done in many ways, and it's important to find a practice that works for you and that you can realistically fit into your schedule. Here are some tips for incorporating mindfulness into your daily routine:

1. Start small: Begin by setting aside just a few minutes each day for mindfulness practice, and gradually increase the amount of time as you become more comfortable.

2. Make it a habit: Try to practice mindfulness at the same time each day, and make it a regular part of your daily routine. This will help to make it a habit and easier to stick to.

3. Find what works for you: Experiment with different mindfulness practices, such as meditation, mindful breathing, or mindful walking, to find what works best for you.

4. Practice mindfulness in daily activities: Incorporate mindfulness into your daily activities such as eating, walking, and doing household chores by paying

attention to your senses and being present in the moment.

5. Use reminders: Use reminders such as alarms or calendar notifications to remind you to practice mindfulness throughout the day.

6. Incorporate mindfulness in your work: Try to be mindful during work by being present and focused on the task at hand, and

taking breaks to breathe and check in with yourself.

Be patient: Remember that mindfulness is a skill that takes practice, and it may take some time to see the benefits. Be patient and don't get discouraged if it's difficult at first.

7. Be kind to yourself: Mindfulness is about being present and non-judgmental. Be kind to yourself and don't get frustrated if your

mind wanders during practice. Simply notice it and gently guide your

Incorporating mindfulness into your daily routine can be done in many ways, here are some examples:

1. Meditation: This can be as simple as taking a few minutes each day to sit quietly and focus on your breath.

2. Mindful breathing: Throughout the day, take a few moments to focus on your breath and bring your attention to the present moment.

3. Mindful listening: When having a conversation with someone, listen attentively and be fully present in the conversation.

4. Mindful walking: Instead of rushing through your walk, pay attention to your surroundings,

the sensation of your feet hitting the ground, and your breath.

5. Mindful eating: Take the time to fully savor and enjoy your food, paying attention to the flavors, textures, and smells.

CHAPTER 7
PUTTING IT ALL TOGETHER

CREATING A PERSONALIZED MIND-BODY BLUEPRINT

Creating a personalized mind-body blueprint is a process of designing an individualized plan that addresses both physical and mental well-being. It involves identifying personal goals and creating a plan to achieve them by taking into account personal preferences, lifestyle, and current physical and mental health. Here are some steps to create a personalized mind-body blueprint:

1. Assess your current physical and mental well-being: Take inventory of your current physical and mental health, including any health conditions or concerns you have. Identify areas of your health that you would like to improve.

2. Identify your goals: Determine what you want to achieve in terms of physical and mental well-being. Set specific, measurable, and realistic goals.

3. Develop a plan: Using your assessment and goals as a guide, develop a plan that includes specific actions to take to achieve your goals. This may include changes to diet, exercise, sleep,

stress management, and other lifestyle habits.

4. Incorporate mindfulness practices: Mindfulness practices such as meditation, yoga, and mindful breathing can be helpful in reducing stress and anxiety, and promoting emotional regulation. Incorporate these practices into your daily routine.

5. Seek professional guidance if needed: If you have specific health concerns or conditions, consider seeking professional guidance from a healthcare provider, nutritionist, or therapist.

6. Review and adjust your plan: Regularly evaluate your progress and make adjustments to your plan as needed. Be flexible and open to making changes as you

learn more about what works best for you.

7. Incorporate self-care practices: Self-care practices such as journaling, reading, and spending time in nature can be beneficial for overall well-being and should be included in your plan.

8. Create a supportive environment: Your environment plays a big role in your overall

well-being. Surround yourself with supportive people, clear out clutter and create a comfortable and inviting space.

Creating a personalized mind-body blueprint is a process of designing an individualized plan that addresses both physical and mental well-being. It is a holistic approach that takes into account the interconnectedness of the mind and body, and recognizes that physical and mental health are closely linked.

Assessing your current physical and mental well-being is the first step in creating a personalized mind-body blueprint. This includes identifying any health conditions or concerns you have, and noting any areas of your health that you would like to improve. This will help to guide the development of your plan and set specific, measurable, and realistic goals.

After identifying your goals, develop a plan that includes specific actions to take to achieve them. This may include changes to diet, exercise, sleep, stress management, and other lifestyle habits. It's important to include a balance of physical activity, healthy eating and stress management techniques in your

from a healthcare provider, nutritionist, or therapist. They can help you to develop a plan that is tailored to your needs and provide guidance and support as you work towards your goals.

STAYING CONNECTED TO YOUR HEALTH AND WELLNESS JOURNEY

Staying committed to your health and wellness journey requires a combination of discipline, motivation, and self-care. It's important to set realistic goals and develop a plan that is tailored to your needs and lifestyle. Creating a schedule and making your health and wellness activities a priority can help to ensure that you make time for them, even when you're busy.

One effective way to stay committed to your health and wellness journey is to find an accountability partner. This can be a friend, family member, or coach who can keep you accountable and motivated. Having someone to share your progress with can be motivating and you can also support each other.

Consistency is key to making progress. Stick to your plan and don't get discouraged if you have setbacks. Instead of getting discouraged, focus on the progress you have made and remind yourself of the reasons why you started your journey. Celebrate small successes along the way, it will help to keep you motivated and focused on your goals.

It's important to be flexible and open to making changes to your plan as needed. Remember that progress is not always linear, and setbacks are a normal part of the process. It's important to stay present in the moment and avoid getting caught up in regrets about the past or worries about the future. Mindfulness practices can help you stay present in the moment and stay focused on your goals.

It's also important to reward yourself for reaching milestones along the way. This will help to keep you motivated and on track. The rewards don't have to be big, it can be something simple like buying a new book or taking a relaxing bath after a hard workout.

Most importantly, take care of yourself and be kind to yourself. Remember that progress takes time and effort, and it's not always easy. Stay committed to your plan, and don't get discouraged if you have setbacks. With patience, consistency, and determination, you can achieve your health and wellness goals.

Staying committed to your health and wellness journey can be challenging, but it's important to keep in mind that progress is not always linear, and setbacks are a normal part of the process. Here are some tips for staying committed to your health and wellness journey:

Set realistic goals: Set specific, measurable, and realistic goals for yourself. These goals should be challenging, but achievable, and should align with your overall health and wellness plan.

1. Create a schedule: Schedule your health and wellness activities into your calendar.

This will help to ensure that you make time for them, even when you're busy.

2. Find an accountability partner: Having someone to share your progress with can be motivating. Find a friend, family member, or a coach to keep you accountable and motivated.

3. Be consistent: Consistency is key to making progress. Stick to your plan and don't get discouraged if you have setbacks.

4. Celebrate small successes: Recognize and celebrate small successes along the way. This will help to keep you motivated and focused on your goals.

5. Be flexible: Be open to making changes to your plan as needed.

Remember that progress is not always linear, and setbacks are a normal part of the process.

6. Focus on the present: Mindfulness practices can help you stay present in the moment and avoid getting caught up in regrets about the past or worries about the future.

7. Reward yourself: Reward yourself for reaching milestones

along the way. This will help to keep you motivated and on track.

Remember, it's important to be kind to yourself and recognize that progress takes time and effort. Stay committed to your plan, and don't get discouraged if you have setbacks. With patience, consistency, and determination, you can achieve your health and wellness goals.

CONCLUSION

'The Mind-Body Blueprint: Unlocking the Secrets to Optimal Health and Wellness' has explored the powerful connection between the mind and body, and how understanding and harnessing this connection can lead to optimal health and wellness. We have discussed the importance of nutrition, physical activity, stress management, and mindfulness in achieving optimal health and wellness, and the benefits of a holistic approach to health and wellness.

By following the steps outlined in this book, you now have the knowledge and tools to create a personalized mind-body blueprint that takes into account your unique needs and preferences. Remember that progress takes time and effort, and it's not always easy, but with patience, consistency, and determination, you can achieve your health and wellness goals.

In addition to the techniques discussed in this book, it's also important to listen to your body, be mindful of your own needs, and take care of yourself. Remember that optimal health and wellness is a lifelong journey and it's important to be kind to yourself and enjoy the process.

Thank you for joining me on this journey towards optimal health and wellness. I hope that this book has been helpful in providing you with the knowledge and tools to improve your physical and mental well-being."